ENERGY DRINKS

THE DAY THEY ALMOST KILLED ME

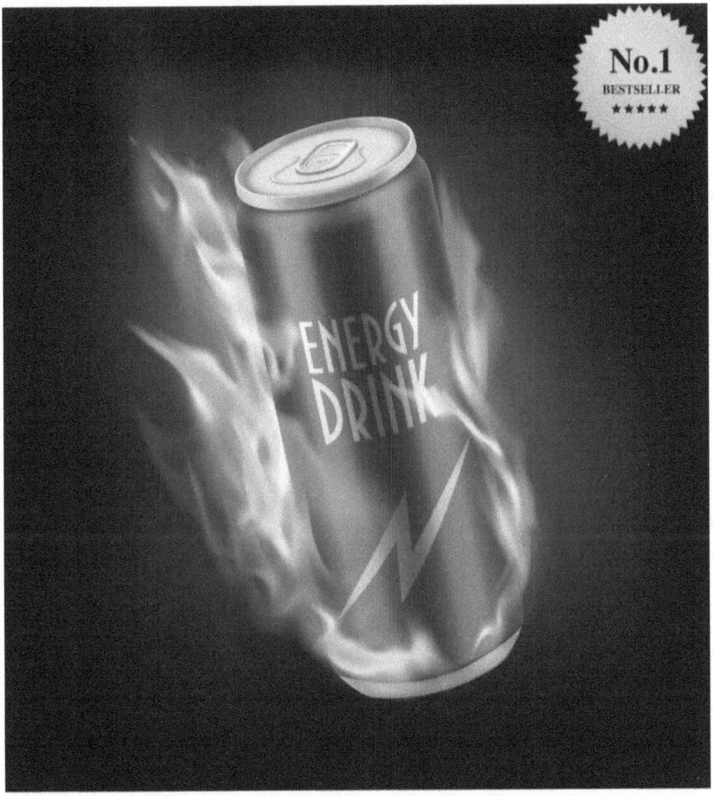

No.1
BESTSELLER
★★★★★

BY AUTHOR: JOE VALENTINE

www.joevalentine.org

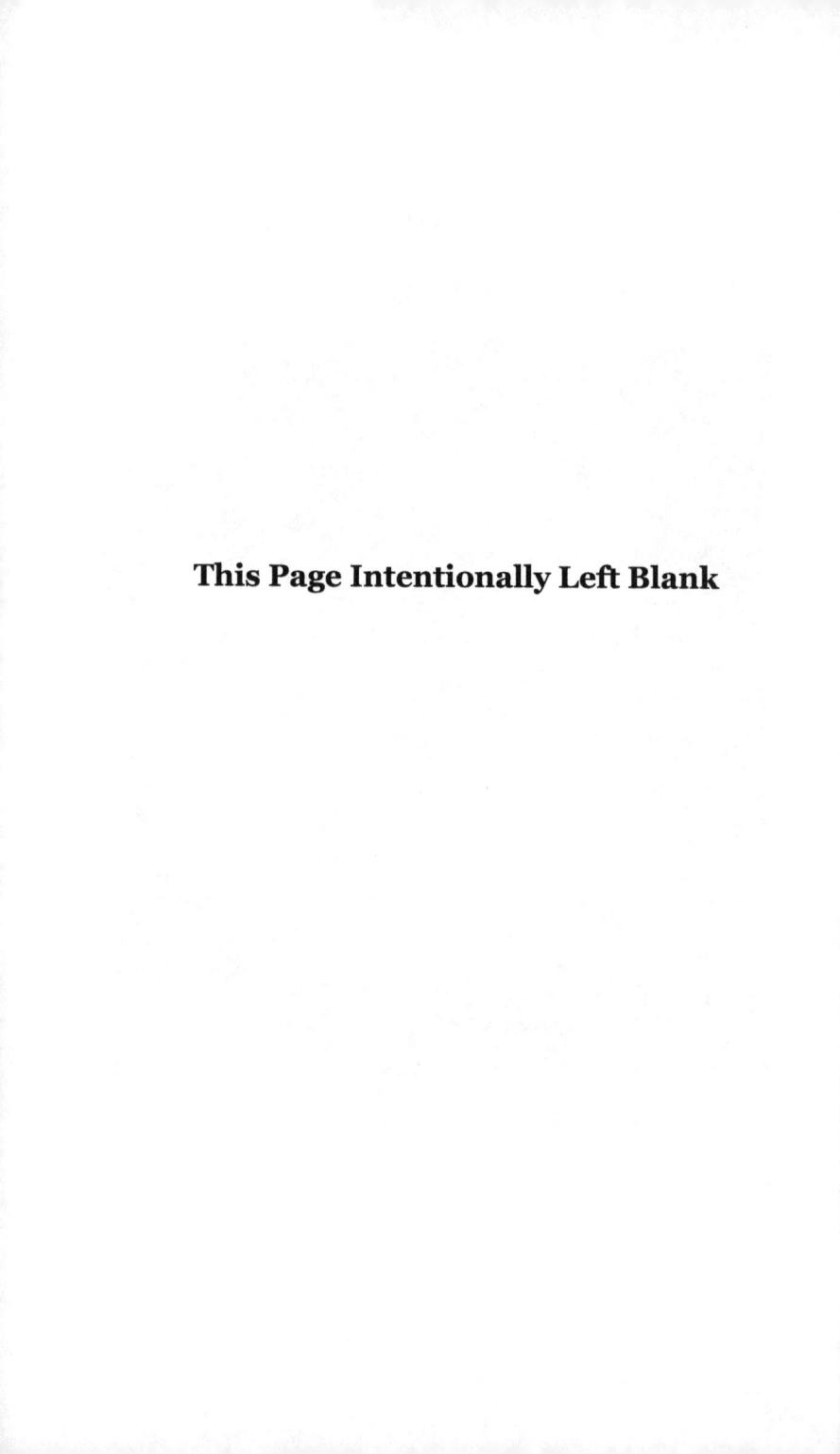

This Page Intentionally Left Blank

Energy Drinks
The Day They Almost Killed Me

The book, "Energy Drinks, The Day They Almost Killed Me" is a great gift for anyone that consumes energy drinks or high doses of caffeine. Knowledge is power, and this book will provide you with information that may save yours, a family member or a friend's life. This book will inspire you to develop healthier habits or encourage you to continue the same bad habits.

A Gift From:_____ Date:_____

(Purchaser of the book)

A Gift To:_____ Date:_____

(Recipient of the book)

Remarks:

_____

_____

_____

Dedication

To parents, husbands, wives, significant others, friends, family members and all who have or know someone who may have been negatively affected by high doses of caffeine or energy drinks:

If it is a loss of life you've experienced, it can't be replaced. If it is a physical or mental change you've experienced, it may not be undone. No one can understand, endure or feel your suffering. Yet, you have the power to prevent someone else from experiencing the pain, taking the path or traveling the road you've already traveled. You can do this by educating others about the possible dangers of substituting high doses of caffeine and energy drinks for sleep and needed energy. With your help we can educate others to make better healthy life choices.

Special Thanks:

Allen Hospital Waterloo, Iowa
Veterans Hospitals everywhere

www.joevalentine.org

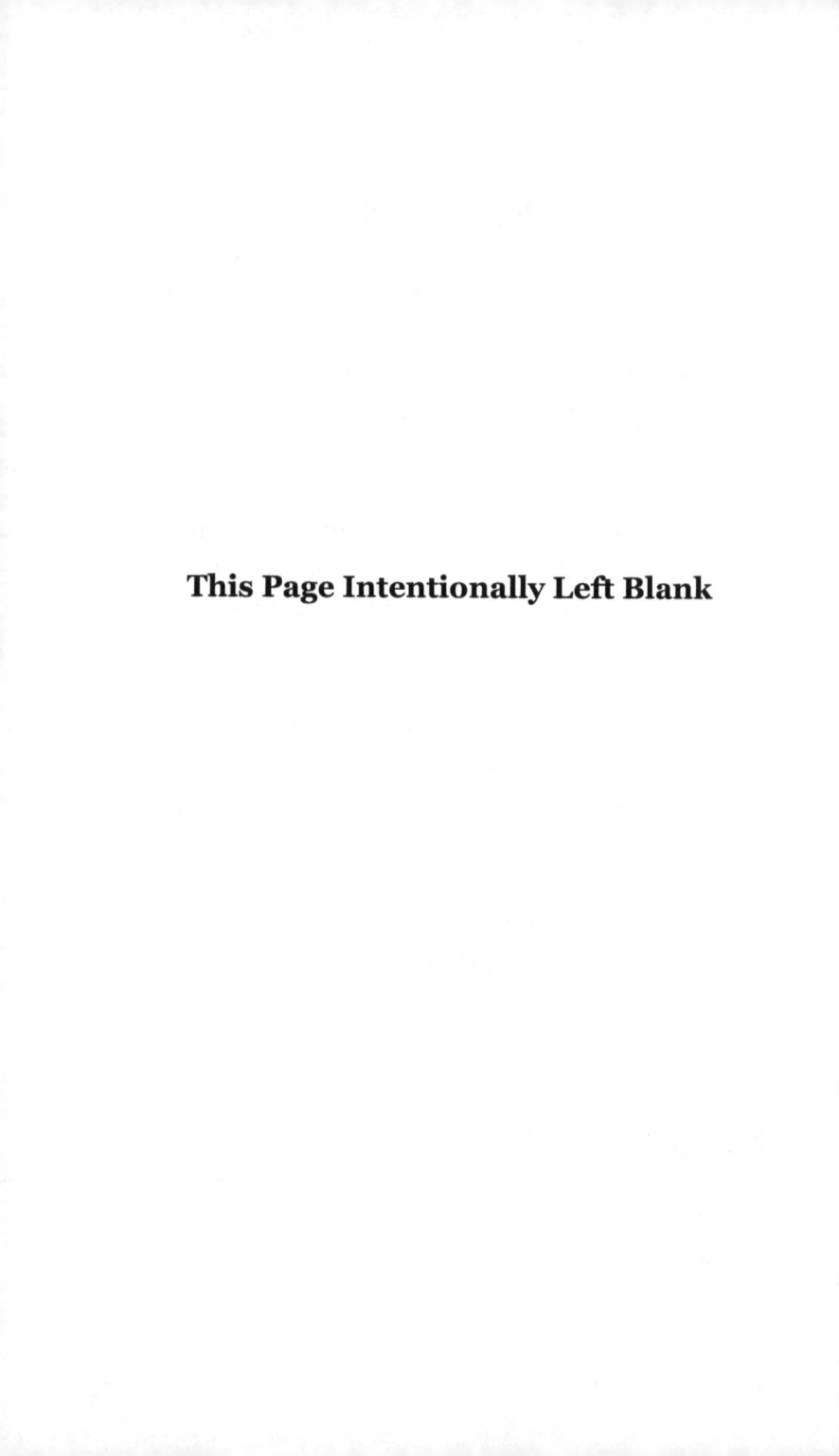
This Page Intentionally Left Blank

Share Your Stories With Us

Post your story on our Facebook page and Subscribe to our YouTube channel. We would love to hear your thoughts, your comments, your testimonials, and your own energy drink and high caffeinated drink stories.

Share your stories: @energydrinkstories

Facebook Page:
https://fb.me/energydrinkstories

Table of Contents

Introduction

Other Books By This Author

__Introduction__

Have you ever drunk an energy drink? Do you know someone who currently drinks energy drinks or high doses of caffeine? Maybe the better question is. Will you or the person you know live to tell your energy drink story? My energy drink experience woke me up to the dangers of energy drinks and consuming high doses of caffeine. The only difference between me and so many others is that I lived to tell you my story. Share this book with everyone you know who consumes energy drinks and high doses of caffeine you may just be saving a life.

Note: Some names have been changed to protect the privacy of the actual participants

Chapter 1

Energy Boost

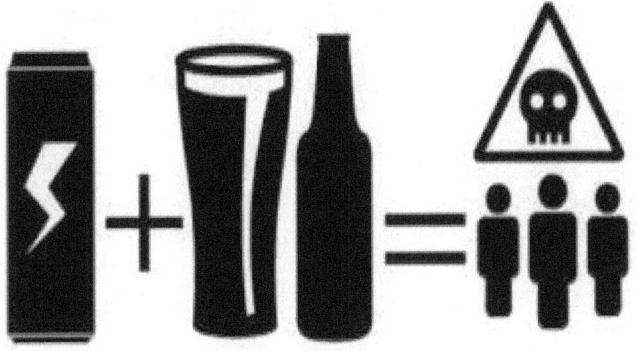

I t was September 22nd three days before my birthday. Death was knocking at my door only I didn't know it. I awoke on the couch with my personal computer still in hand, literally still in my hands.

It had been a long night.

I worked my way through the night diligently while, often recalling my grandfather Delmar's voice in my head to keep me motivated, to keep me woke, to keep me going.

Let's go, the Sun is up.

There is work, to be done.

We can't rest until our work is done.

Work hard, and don't stop until the job is done.

My grandfather would repeat these sayings to my brother and I every morning during our summer vacations in the deep south, Mississippi.

I learned how to work hard, how to work long, how to work tirelessly by eating the right foods and getting adequate sleep.

Somewhere along the way I lost sight of this.

I was never taught to substitute sleep with liquid energy boosters that became a learned behavior I taught myself as an adult.

This particular night, I worked and worked until my eyelids could take no more.

I fought it as long as I could.

I was determined to get it done.

Sleep finally got the best of me.

I fell asleep while working on the new mental health company we launched a few months earlier. I did it was the last thought to myself as I entered the realm of sleep.

I achieved the American dream of creating generational wealth, but at what cost.

Unbeknown to me, five hours later generational wealth and businesses would be the least important thing on my mind.

I drunk something I thought was helping me.

I drunk something I had drunk hundreds of times before.

I drunk something I thought was perfectly safe.

How would I know something I've drunk numerous times before would almost cost me my life?

I awoke a few hours later from what I thought was a short nap.

Immediately upon awaking I noticed I felt kind of weird.

Something wasn't right.

I heard a loud noise coming from inside of me.

I turned my head and looked left but saw nothing.

I looked right but came up with the same result, nothing.

I still heard the noise coming from within.

I looked down.

It was my chest.

My chest was jumping uncontrollably.

What the heck?

What's wrong with me?

From my perspective, it looked like a bad rendition of an animated sci-fi film from the early 1960's. The view looked so unreal, so fake I turned my head to look away as if what I just saw wasn't happening.

Still hearing the noise, I turned my head back in the direction of my chest to do a double take. The second view was just as bad as the first view.

My chest was still moving and jumping out of control.

I quickly reached for my Asthma inhaler.

I was sure I was having a massive Asthma attack.

I quickly gave myself two puffs of the bright yellow inhaler.

I wanted to do everything possible to head off this asthma attack.

My chest beat uncontrollably, speeding up a bit.

I sat up on the couch, frantically.

Maybe if I do some work, calm down and take my mind off of my chest, it will go away.

I pushed in the flashing power button on my personal computer as it sat undisturbed.

I desperately wanted to ignore whatever it was I was experiencing.

I gazed outside the living room window from the couch.

It was early in the a.m.; the birds were chirping, and the sun was just starting to make its way up over the horizon in the east.

Oh well, my chest will stop pounding sooner or later.

Back at it.

It's time to get to work.

I reopened spreadsheets and word documents I was working on prior to falling asleep.

I started working diligently as if nothing at all was going on.

I tried and tried to ignore the strange awkward feeling I was having in my chest.

I ignored the pounding for an hour and a half.

Finally, I could not ignore the loud internal sound anymore.

The sound agitated me.

I looked down again at my chest to verify I wasn't dreaming.

Sure, enough my chest was still jumping.

This time my chest was jumping like a bunch of jumping beans jumping off the floor.

Something happened.

I started seeing not from my own eyes rather I was outside of my own body looking away from myself.

It was as if I had an out of body experience or what some may call an epiphany.

In my moment of delusion, I found myself standing in front of my coffee table instead of being seated on the living room sofa as I was in reality.

I found myself to be levitating and floating in the air upwards towards the ceiling.

I floated a short distance to the window and gazed out of it.

Moments later I saw the top of a shaved bald head peering through the window while someone was talking on his cell phone.

The individual was starring right at me only they did not see me.

In my hallucination the man peering through the window spoke to someone on the phone.

I haven't seen Joe in days.

His family wanted me to stop by and check on him.

I quickly realized in this dream state I was apparently missing.

The gentleman peeking through the window continued speaking into his cell phone as he walked away from the window towards the side of the house.

I heard the same voice utter; I'm going to kick in his back door if necessary.

The man kicked in the back door and wondered through my home.

He found me non-responsive seated upright on the couch, dead with an energy drink not too far from me.

Just as quick as the epiphany started, it ended.

In a split second I transitioned back to my current reality, seated on the couch.

The vision scared the hell out of me.

I quickly realized I needed to get myself to the hospital.

My chest was still beating uncontrollably for nearly three hours now.

I started speaking to myself.

I have to get to the hospital.

I have to get to the hospital right now.

Let me get up and drive myself to Iowa City!

I quickly dressed myself.

Nobody but me would think to pack my personal computer so I could continue to work while the doctor was checking me out, but I did.

I unplugged the laptop.

I grabbed a number of my files I was working on.

I jumped into my Cadillac Escalade truck enroute to the VA Hospital nearly two hours away.

I drove down Martin Luther King Boulevard at a steady fast rate.

I approached downtown nearing the intersection at Franklin Street.

My corporate office was located only two blocks up ahead.

I was stopped by a red traffic light at the corner of Franklin Street.

This gave me an opportune time to think.

While sitting there waiting for the light to turn green I tried to ignore my beating chest.

I found myself thinking about all the items I needed out of my office.

I wasn't focused on getting better I was focused on completing the necessary paperwork for the expansion of our new mental health office in Des Moines.

I spoke to myself to take my mind off my heart.

I need more paperwork from the office just in case the emergency room is crowded.

It might take all day!

You know how long those emergency rooms take.

My chest was still beating like a drummer boy was playing it out of control.

Let me call Stacy.

Stacy was a Registered Nurse and a supervisor on the heart floor at one of our local hospitals in the city, Allen Hospital.

Stacy had been a long-time childhood friend and our families knew each other well.

We grew up in the same neighborhood.

I grabbed my cell phone from the inside pocket of my long black trench coat.

It took a few seconds for me to find Stacy's phone number but when I did, I put it to good use.

I called Stacy's phone only to receive communication from her voicemail, but I left no message. It's early Saturday morning she's probably still asleep.

In normal circumstances, I would not have called Stacy back, but this wasn't normal circumstances at all.

I called Stacy's cell phone again.

It rung and it rung.

Stacy finally answered.

Boy, what are you doing calling my phone this early in the morning?

Hey, I have a question for you.

What is it?

It better be a good question since you are calling me this early on my day off.

It is.

My chest has been beating like crazy since 4:30 this morning.

What do you think it is?

What............ Stacy replied!!!!

Say again!

I could hear it in her voice.

Stacy took a deep breath.

She jumped right into nurse's mode.

Can you check your heart rate for me?

No, it's beating to fast I don't think I can count

the beats.

Where are you?

I'm in my truck, stopped at a red traffic light at

the corner of Franklin Street and Martin

Luther

King Boulevard.

I'm headed to my office to get some paperwork

and then I'm driving to Iowa City to the

VA Hospital.

Boy, have you lost your damn mind?

I replied what are you talking about?

Joe get your butt up to the hospital, right away!

You don't have time to drive an hour and half to the VA Hospital!

I want to go to the VA Hospital then I won't get a bill.

Joe really?

Stop being cheap and get your butt (explicit language) up to Allen Hospital, right now!

You think so?

You think this is that serious?

Yes, it is that darn (explicit language) serious!

Get your butt (explicit language) up to that hospital right now!

The streetlight turned green.

Stacy was still yelling in my ear.

Get your butt (explicit language) up to the emergency room right now.

Reluctantly, my plans to stop by my office and travel to the VA Hospital in Iowa City changed. I made a right turn onto Franklin Street and headed in the direction of the nearest emergency room.

Stacy convinced me her way was best.

Chapter 2

The Flash

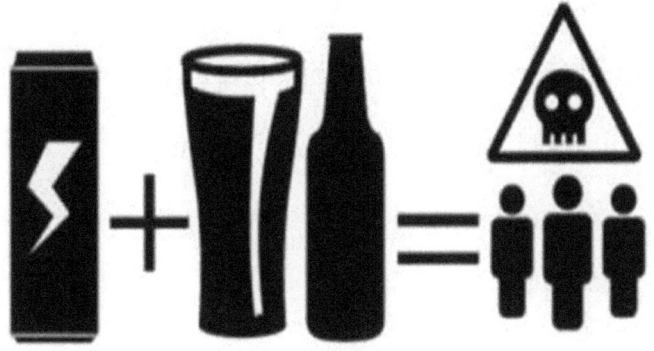

Emergency room was my destination. I arrived at Allen Hospital emergency room in a flash.

I parked my truck in the parking lot as if I would be right back out in a few minutes.

I still had little idea of what was truly happening to me.

I opened the truck door.

I couldn't forget my laptop as I reached back in to grab it.

I walked casually into the emergency room entrance as if nothing was wrong with me.

An intake nurse seated behind the desk in her blue scrubs looked up and smiled at me.

I approached her as she spoke.

How can I help you?

Well, my heart has been beating fast since about 4:30 a.m. this morning.

The nurse froze.

She looked at me as if she was in shock of what I just said.

The nurses mouth gapped open and was stuck in a wide-open position.

Her eyebrows were fixed in a high arch.

Time froze for a split second as I waited for the nurse to respond.

Suddenly the nurse quickly went into action.

She snatched the telephone sitting in front of her on the desk.

The nurse called back to the interior of the emergency room I imagine.

Moments later, the two slate gray doors behind her quickly swung open.

A nurse dressed in light blue scrubs as if she was preparing for surgery rushed through the doors pushing a wheelchair straight towards me.

She spoke hastily to the receptionist nurse seated at the desk.

Where is the patient?

This is him standing.

Sir take a seat here!

We are going to take good care of you.

I smiled slightly as if to introduce myself to the nurse.

I'm okay I believe, it's not that serious.

We will be the judge of that, sir.

We will take good care of you and figure out what is going on.

Please sit here.

I slowly sat down in the wheelchair, clutching my laptop bag as if nothing was wrong with me.

Quickly the emergency room nurse spun me around.

The gigantic gray double doors opened quickly.

We were off like a racehorse out of the gate.

We headed back deep into the emergency room at a very fast pace.

If we were outside the hospital the nurse probably would have been ticketed at her rate of travel.

I thought to myself it's not that serious.

As we traveled down the hallway more nurses and doctors dropped what they were doing and jumped in line behind us.

Everybody followed closely behind the wheelchair as if we were a part of a traveling caravan traveling across a vast desert.

We quickly made it to a room with an empty bed at the end of the hallway.

The nurse pushing my wheelchair snatched my laptop out of my hand all while speaking.

I'm going to place your laptop over here in the corner, in a safe place.

The next thing I knew multiple nurses helped me out of the wheelchair and onto a hospital gurney.

I looked up only to see more people running into the room with each passing second.

Multiple nurses began stripping clothes from me.

Other nurses attempted to calm me down with soothing words, words of confidence.

I was confused.

I was confused because I assumed not much was wrong with me.

I only thought I needed a breathing treatment and some asthma medications.

Two nurses began to peel off adhesive stickers.

The nurses attached sticky adhesives to my body.

The next thing I knew, I had several multiple colored wires crisscrossing all over my body.

I lifted my head from the hospital gurney.

I wanted to see what was going on.

I started feeling a little weird, more weirder than I was already feeling.

A nurse quickly grabbed the nearest phone and began to scream out code colors and a room number over the intercom.

The sound blared out over my head up above me.

The sound filled the entire room.

It was a mad house as more doctors and more nurses rushed into the room.

I was oblivious as to what was going on.

A male nurse approached the right side of the gurney I was lying on.

He stood next to my head, leaned over and grabbed my hand.

The male nurse spoke to me.

Joe, that's your name isn't it?

Yes!

It's going to be okay.

What are you talking about?

Your heart is in overdrive, but don't worry we're going to slow it back down.

We will take good care of you.

Who drove you here?

I did?

You're kidding me?

Wow!

I don't even understand how you are conscious and talking to me right now?

What do you mean?

What's going on with me?

Don't worry about it.

You just worry about getting better, okay?

Is there a wife or immediate relatives we can call for you?

No, I'm divorced, and all my relatives and immediate family members are either in Mississippi or on their way to Mississippi for our family reunion this weekend.

I was supposed to leave Iowa last night to drive down to the family reunion, but I changed my mind at the last minute.

There has to be somebody here we can call for you.

Yes, there is!

Call my childhood friend, my business partner, Rodney.

He can contact my mother and brothers for me if necessary.

What's Rodney's number Joe?

I provided the nurse with Rodney's cell phone number.

Right at that moment fear jumped all over me.

For the first time, I was scared.

My mental health background kicked in.

I began to positive self-talk myself as if I was a mental health patient in a room alone with a doctor.

To me the room went silent.

I looked down at my chest.

It was jumping, jumping faster and faster.

My heart was determined to exist outside of my body.

I began to talk to myself even more.

Specifically, I talked directly to my heart.

I lifted my head from the gurney table.

I lowered my chin and gazed down at my chest.

Me and my heart had to have a direct conversation with one another.

Slow down!

Slow down!

Please slow down!

I told myself this over and over.

I wanted full control of my body, but my body wasn't cooperating.

For the first time the idea of heart problems crept into my head.

Fear was trying to take over and I was refusing
to let it.

I thought I could correct my physical problem
by merely continuing to address the issue
directly to my chest.

So, I continued with my rubbish.

Slow down heart.

Slow down.

The more I attempted to calm my heart the
more it continued to beat out of control.

For the first time in my life, I realized I wasn't
truly in control of my own body.

I panicked.

I became very, very scared even more scared
than before.

I was having a heart attack.

The male nurse holding my hand saw the terror in my eyes.

Nothing up to this point had been more terrifying to me in my life.

The male nurse tried to comfort me.

I could see he was doing his best to prevent an all-out cataclysm.

Don't worry about it, Joe.

Everything is going to be all right.

The less you worry, the better you will be.

Think good thoughts, no bad thoughts.

Let's talk, you and me?

Do you have any children?

Of course, I have children I thought to myself, but no words left my mouth.

I never answered the question.

I was terrified.

I was frightened and in awe of all that was happening around me.

I was bewildered by the massive number of people frantically moving around the room.

Hands on and hands off continued to touch me one after another.

Sometimes I could feel multiple hands touching me and working on me simultaneously.

A Doctor pushed his way through the crowded room and approached the right side of the bed.

The Doctor stepped around the male nurse who was still holding my hand.

I turned my head gazing at the doctor as he approached me.

The doctor had in hand what appeared to be a gigantic syringe full of a milk looking substance.

Hi, I am Doctor Johnson.

I am the Doctor that will be taking care of you today.

I have some medicine in this needle, I'm going to shoot into your arm.

The medicine is going to slow your heart rate down.

What is it Doc?

It's called Propofol.

I responded promptly.

Propofol?

Isn't that the sh--t that killed Michael Jackson?

The room became silent.

It seemed like the entire emergency room stopped moving all at once.

The Doctor eyes grew big and he tried to hold back his smile, but he couldn't.

The Doctor erupted into laughter.

That's the first time anyone has ever said that to me!

But you are right!

Yes, it is the same stuff that killed Michael Jackson.

Well, I don't want it!

You have to take it!

You have no other choice at this point!

It's just going to slow your heart rate and put you to sleep.

That's the problem DOC!

I don't want to go to sleep.

I might not wake up!

Son, if you don't take this medicine you won't wake up!

You have to take it now!

It's just going to put you to sleep and slow your heart rate down some.

Okay, Doc!

A nurse listening to the doctor and listening to my confrontational dialogue grabbed me by the arm.

The nurse held it tightly as the doctor prepared to inject the needle.

The doctor leaned over towards me, quickly spotted a vein and injected the Propofol into my arm.

Seconds passed as the doctor watched and observed the heart rate monitor.

This is strange!

I've never had to give anyone two doses of Propofol!

Son, I'm going to give you another shot of Propofol.

What?

Are you serious?

Yes, I'm very serious.

We have to get your heart under control.

The doctor quickly instructed a nurse to get another syringe of Propofol.

Seconds passed by as time was of the utmost importance.

The nurse handed the doctor a new syringe full of the lifesaving or life ending drug. Without further warning the doctor quickly injected the second dose of Propofol into my arm.

A few seconds later, I was unconscious.

I don't know how long I was out.

I don't know what exactly happened in my brief absence.

Upon opening my eyes, I saw a familiar face next to my bed.

It was Rodney.

Rodney was seated in a chair pulled up close to the left side of my bed.

Rodney spoke.

Don't say anything little brother, keep your strength.

God has you; you're going to be okay.

I spoke with the doctors and they told me everything.

I've already called your brother in St. Louis.

He has already called your mother, Mrs. Shirley and your brother Scott.

I spoke with your mother and told her I will keep them updated on your progress.

I lifted my head from the hospital bed.

I looked down at my chest to see what was going on.

I no longer heard the pounding of drums as if I was a kid at the drive-in theater watching "King Kong" on the big screen appearing for the first time out of the shadows of the jungle to get his bride.

I no longer felt the throbbing and pounding coming from within.

Oh, I felt pain alright, but it was a different kind of pain.

This pain was not coming from the inside of me but rather from the outside of me this time.

I felt it and even saw some reddish looking impressions on my chest.

The expressions on my face said I wanted some answers and the doctor knew it.

The doctor gazed down at his clipboard, but he felt obliged to give me some answers, so he did.

Don't worry about the chest pain from the bruises they will go away soon over the next few days.

We had to heat you up just a little bit.

We had to put the pedals on your chest to get your heart back in rhythm.

I laid my head back down in a bit of surprise.

I had never had that happen to me before.

The morning was starting off with a day full of FIRST!

I was deep in my own thoughts.

What just happened I asked myself?

I tried and tried but I could not recall anything.

I couldn't remember anything from the moment the second injection of Propofol entered my veins.

I only remember opening my eyes from complete silence and complete darkness.

Was this what it is like to be dead, I quietly thought to myself.

How you feeling little bro?

You need me to do anything?

No, I'm good.

What are you doing here Rodney?

How are you doing?

I'm good thank you for asking.

I'm here to help out my brother.

Thank you, Rodney, for coming.

No problem, we from City View that's what we
do, we look out for one another.

I had known Rodney most of my life.

I 've known his brother, his sisters, his mother
and his father.

Not only had I known them, but our
neighborhood was a pretty close-knit place.

It was a neighborhood in those days where if a parent saw you doing something wrong, they corrected you on the spot.

Most of the time that correction was accompanied by a call or personal visit to your parent's front door.

There was no shortage of words in those days, no shortage of words of other parents telling on you for anything you did disrespectful or wrong.

Ironically, one summer day my mother caught Rodney taking some apples from an apple tree. The owner Charlie Ray told all the neighborhood kids over and over that his apple trees in his yard were off limits.

This was and interaction Rodney would never forget.

Mom told Rodney that day to get out of Charlie Ray's apple tree's all while scolding him that he knew better.

Minutes later, Mom marched right down to Rodney's mother's house and told all she knew as if a bank robbery had occurred.

Mrs. Nettie did not take it to kindly that her son was taking apples that didn't belong to him.

Our neighborhood was a neighborhood back then that understood the old saying, "It takes a village to raise a child."

City View was a place when the streetlights came on, the kids all scattered and scrambled to get inside.

This was one friend I could count on.

It took me a minute to remember where I was at.

It took a minute to remember all that happened to me today.

Thanks for coming Rodney

Boy, what are you talking about!

You know we take care of our own.

Me being here was God sent.

It was meant by God.

Rodney nor I could truly comprehend that statement, but we would understand it in the hours yet to come.

We didn't know but, God already knew what was yet to transpire.

God placed Rodney right where he needed to be that morning at Allen Hospital instead of out of the state on a business excursion.

Brother, God is good.

I was supposed to be out of the state on a business trip this morning.

I woke up and cancelled my trip early this morning for some reason.

For some reason, I felt I should stay around home today.

I felt I had to take care of something here this weekend instead of leaving.

God already knew I was supposed to be here with you, little brother.

I responded.

Thank the LORD he kept you around today.

My entire family are in or headed to

Mississippi for our annual family reunion, my

maternal grandmother's side of the family.

I was supposed to leave yesterday morning

myself.

I changed my mind at the last minute and

decided not to go at all this year.

Rodney, think about it.

If I had left yesterday, I would have died on the

highway this morning driving down south to

Mississippi.

God is always right on time.

Thank you, Jesus, for sparing me and giving

me more time here on Earth.

Amen brother.

God does not make any mistakes!

Get you some rest little brother.

I'm just going to step outside the room for a minute and call your mother and brothers.

I will give them an update on everything.

Rodney stepped outside the room for a few minutes.

I glared up at the bright lights shinning down on me from the hospital gurney I was stretched out over.

I reached over to my left in an effort to get another hospital blanket.

I was freezing.

Despite this, I could not find one.

A nurse walked in and I quickly went into action.

Do you have any more blankets?

Yes, I will bring you some warm blankets in a few minutes.

How are you feeling?

I'm doing okay, just really cold.

You seem to be doing much better.

The nurse leaned over to check my vitals on the EKG machine hooked up to me.

The nurse made some notations on her clip board.

I will be back in a moment.

I'm going to grab those warm blankets for you.

Okay.

I was out of harm's way and focused on getting warm.

Rodney made his entrance back into the room a few moments later.

I just spoke with your mother.

Mrs. Shirley is worried sick about you.

She asked me what happened.

I told her you had some heart problems, but you are doing find now.

Thank you.

I don't want her worried about me.

One of the doctor's helping during my heart catastrophe made his way back into the room just as I started closing my eyes.

How is it going Joe?

I feel good Doc.

Where is the other doctor that gave me the shot?

He is with some other needy patients.

Since we have you stable now, I figured you would want to see my pretty face.

Will he be back in to talk to me?

No, his shift is ending soon so I will be taking over.

How are you feeling now?

Any light headedness?

Any vision problems?

Any more racing of the heart feelings?

No, doc I'm feeling pretty good.

Okay.

Tell me about your week.

Any history of heart troubles in your family?

No, doc!

No heart problems that I am aware of in my family at all.

It seems like your heart was under a lot of stress.

Anything you did out of the ordinary this week?

No, doc.

I just worked like I've been doing and running off four to five hours of nightly sleep.

You said four to five hours of sleep?

Yes, doc.

I've been sleeping four to five hours nightly for years ever since I was in and left the United States Marine Corp.

That's not good!

You must try and get eight hours or more of sleep per night.

Doc, I taught myself how to run off four to five hours of sleep from my days of pulling all night duties staying up playing war games in the field in the Marine Corp.

If I get four to five hours of sleep, I feel refreshed and great when I wake up.

Back to this week.

Did you take anything or drink excessive coffee this week?

I drink coffee every now and then.

Oh yeah!

I was tired when I left Des Moines yesterday evening.

I stopped, gassed up, I grabbed some energy drinks and drove home.

My day was pretty typical.

You're kidding me!

ENERGY DRINKS!!!

Yes!

I had a few energy drinks.

Son, energy drinks can kill you!

Energy drinks are one of the worst things in the world for the heart.

Those drinks should be illegal!

Energy drinks should be outlawed for sale!

What!!!!!!!!

Should be outlawed?????

What are you talking about doc?

Energy drinks are bad for you.

Really?????

Yes!

For the life of me, I don't know how the government still allows those things to be sold to the general public.

They should be illegal in my opinion.

Doc, you're kidding me, right?

Absolutely not!

Son, do you understand what you're putting into your mouth?

Do you know what the contents are in energy drinks?

Son, you were drinking liquid cocaine in a bottle!

That stuff shouldn't be sold anywhere in the world, especially in the United States!

Silence was in the room for a few seconds.

I laid there staring at the doctor, perplexed.

In astonishment I thought to myself, how could this be.

If it's that bad doc, how can they get away with the sale of energy drinks then?

If you made eighty million dollars a year and you only paid out ten million dollars a year wouldn't you say that is good business?

Yes, but what are they paying the ten million for?

To the families of those that died drinking energy drinks.

What????

Sad but true.

Millions of dollars a year in profit to those tycoons outweigh a measly life of someone they don't know.

I'm going to leave you here to rest.

I will be back to check on you in an hour or so.

If you need anything or if there is an emergency, hit the nurses call button on the side of your bed.

We here at Allen are here to take care of you.

Okay, doc.

Rodney sat in his chair next to my bed as though he was a lion protecting his cub.

You just don't find many of these types of friendships and acts of caring in this day and age.

I started closing my eyes when Rodney said.

Get you some sleep little bro.

I will be here when you wake up.

I fell into a deep sleep without responding to his words.

Minutes passed by, so I thought.

I awoke just as fast as I fell asleep.

In reality, two or three hours had by passed.

I looked to my left and Rodney was still seated in the same spot.

His back was facing me.

He was sitting quietly texting on his phone with an occasional glance up at the television mounted in the ceiling.

Hey brother, you still here?

Shoot!

I'm not going anywhere.

God meant for me to be here today so I'm going to follow his instructions.

I'm going to listen to his voice.

During our brief talk a doctor I did not recognize entered the room.

How is it going Joe?

Doc, I feel great.

I believe I only needed a little bit of rest.

Okay, we will see.

Let me check your vitals and your heartbeat.

The doctor took a few steps towards the EKG machine.

He started reading the numbers on it.

He pulled out his stethoscope and placed it over my heart.

Speechlessness was in the air for few seconds as Rodney and I awaited the exam results.

Sounds good.

You are doing much better.

Great!

I should be able to go home in a couple of hours then!

We will see after a few more hours of observations.

Come on doc!

I feel great!

I have a lot of work to do with this new company I just started.

We will look at all the possibilities in a few hours.

If you're steadily improving after a couple more hours, I may let you go home.

I gazed over and looked towards Rodney for moral support for going home but support from him at this moment was not to be.

Rodney had a look on his face.

It was a look I had seen all too often in the neighborhood growing up.

His facial expression was a mixture between confusion, concern and anger all three faces split into one.

Rodney couldn't hold his peace any longer and he spoke up.

No!

No!

No, sir!

Doc, unless you can tell me this man only had a common cold there is absolutely no way you should be considering letting him go home today.

Joe!

My brother!

We're both from City View!

If you think you are going home today, we both will be fighting up in here!

Doc!

I know you didn't just tell this man; he can go home today!

I know I just didn't hear that!

I know you didn't mean what you just said doc!

Doc, you need to keep my brother overnight.

You need to keep him at least for a twenty-four-hour observation.

Joe, I think your friend is right!

We will keep you for a few more days.

Really????

You can't be serious!

Oh, I'm very serious!

I will call upstairs and get you admitted into the hospital.

Rodney in agreement spoke.

Amen!

Now you're talking doc!

I laid there in the bed confused, like what just happened.

I was almost out of here I concluded in quietude.

I only could think about the enormous amount of work I had to get done.

Unbelievable!

A team will be in shortly to take you over to the hospital side plus we have great hospital food!

They will get you settled in your hospital room.

I will visit you tomorrow, but another doctor will be assigned to care for you going forward.

I was pissed.

Whatever you say doc.

I guess, I have no choice but to be around.

The doctor walked out of the room chuckling under his breath with a comical smile on his face.

My face on the other hand was quite the opposite.

I just wanted out of here.

I wanted to be back in my office.

I have no time to be stopping the progress of my life, my children's lives, my grandchildren and my family members lives.

It was and is my belief God granted me certain skills to make a positive difference in their lives.

Rodney started talking as if he knew I was in deep thought about something.

Little bro, work can wait!

Anything else you have going on in your head can wait.

It all can wait until you are better.

You're going to be all right!

God doesn't make no mistakes!

God is going to bring you through this and provide you with a story to tell!

We are speaking it into existence!

We are claiming it!

Now, let's say a prayer.

Rodney stood up from the chair he was seated in.

He leaned in and over my bed.

He grabbed my left hand, closed his eyes and bowed his head.

I followed suit by closing my eyes and bowed my head as much as I could.

Rodney prayed.

Father!

We come to you asking for your mercy.

Father, we come to you asking for your grace.

Father, if it is your will.

Father, if it is your plan.

Father heal my brothers' body, spirit and soul in the name of Jesus.

Amen!

Amen!

See, I told you not to worry!

God's got this!

You're going to be all right little bro.

A few nurses entered my temporary staging area just as we finished up our worship and prayer solemnity.

Hi, Joe.

We are here to gather your belongings and transport you up to your room over in the hospital wing of Allen Hospital.

Hi, I begrudgingly replied.

This Page Intentionally Left Blank

Chapter 3

The Stay

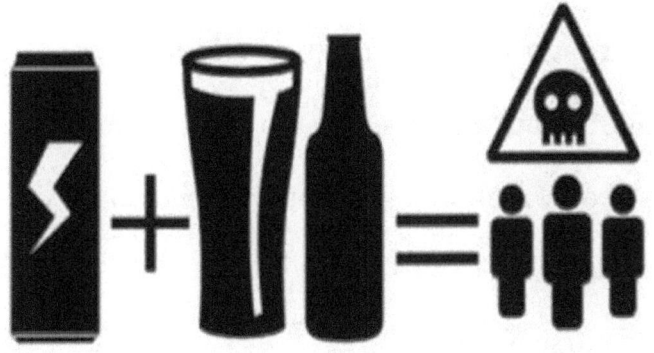

www.joevalentine.org

The nurses approached my bedside and began to gather cords, unhook machines, secure side railings etc.... It took a few minutes, but we were already to go. Rodney helped by grabbing some of my personal belongings.

The nurse became vocal.

Ok, Joe.

We have everything.

We're going to unlock the wheels on your bed and roll you down to the elevator now.

Once we are in the elevator, we will take you up to the third floor on the hospital side.

I nodded my head in agreement.

Even though if it was up to me, I would be sitting behind the steering wheel of my Cadillac Escalade truck driving enroute to my home.

Rodney stepped outside of the emergency room.

He had all my personal belongings in his hands.

The nurses pushed the bed forward and out of my current room.

We were off.

It had been six hours since my heart had raced out of control.

I was in the clear and feeling pretty good in my own self-reflection.

I laid back on the bed with little concern for what already transpired.

The ceiling lights above zoomed by as we made our way down the hall.

In a twinkling, we approached the elevators.

With the push of a button the elevator doors opened.

Rodney, the nurses and I boarded the elevator.

The elevators doors closed just as fast as they opened.

Stillness was in the air as the elevator music I was expecting was not present.

I looked forward to getting settled in my new room.

I looked forward to it not for the reasons you may think.

My new-found philosophy was one just implemented a short time ago, "the faster I get settled, the faster I could get the heck out of here!"

Ding!

The elevator bell rung letting us know we've reached our destination, the third floor.

The doors opened.

Rodney stepped out of the elevator first.

Shortly thereafter, the nurses began to push the emergency room bed out of the elevator.

Abruptly, I felt a hard thump in my chest.

I looked down troubled.

Thump, thump!

It did it again.

Thump, thump!

Swiftly, my heart started racing again.

I looked normal on the outside but inside I knew something was wrong.

Not a nurse knew what was going on internally.

I had to say something.

Nurse, somethings wrong!

Help me!

What's that you say Joe?

Something is wrong!

Please, please!

Help me!

My heart is beating fast again!

Cold blue!

Cold blue!

Rodney spoke and attempted to provide some words of encouragement.

Calm down Joe, let them take care of you.

The nurse interrupted.

Sir, you must step away from him, so we can work on him.

Rodney started stepping away from the gurney.

I noticed nurses and doctors running everywhere again.

Doctors came out of the woodworks from every corner of the hospital.

Everyone was packed into the hallway.

There was not enough time to roll me down the hall into a room.

Rodney put some words into action to comfort me.

Brother, I'm going to be right over here.

Don't worry!

Don't have any fear!

God has you!

Don't worry!

Suddenly, I saw another familiar face.

A male nurse ran up to the side of my bed.

It was the nice male nurse from the emergency room downstairs.

He grabbed my hand and started talking.

I just knew it was you when I heard the code over the intercom.

Don't worry Joe, we're going to take good care of you.

Stay calm and think about good things.

This time was different.

The first time this occurred I wasn't scared.

I didn't know what was happening prior to getting to the emergency room so some fear set in but this time I'm terrified.

I'm scared beyond belief.

This time I knew my heart was in A-fib as one of the doctor's downstairs called it.

Fear raced through my mind.

I found myself talking to myself again.

Come on Joe, calm down!

Calm down, Joe!

The male nurse started giving me instructions.

A nurse is going to give you another injection to calm you down.

Joe do you remember the last injection of the milky looking stuff.

Yes.

This is it again and it will also slow your heart rate down.

I glanced to my right side and saw a needle being injected into my I.V.

Mere seconds later I was out and unconscious.

I don't know how long I was out this time.

I woke up feeling groggy.

My chest was hurting again.

I imagine they had to heat me up again by putting the pedals on my chest to get my heart back into rhythm.

This time I dare not ask why my chest was hurting.

I glanced around the room to see my whereabouts.

I was in an unfamiliar room.

We made it into my assigned hospital room.

I looked to my left to see a familiar face seated next to my bed.

Rodney was seated at my bedside watching television.

Hey, big bro.

What happened?

How you feeling little brother?

I'm feeling pretty good.

I prayed for you again and I claimed it!

God said, you're going to be alright.

Thank you, brother.

I can't thank you enough for being here.

Man, what are you talking about?

God wanted me here that's why he cancelled my business flight this morning.

God knew I was supposed to be here with you.

Get you some rest.

Go back to sleep.

I will be here when you wake up.

Extremely exhausted I was.

I was dead tired and closed my eyes to enter the world of sleep.

I awoke to find four hours had passed on the wall clock in front of me.

I glanced to my left again and sure enough Rodney was still seated in his same position.

Two nurses entered the room right at that time.

Hi, Joe.

Were just going to check your monitors and make sure everything is ok.

How are you feeling?

I feel good now that I am rested.

Okay, that's good news.

Your vitals have been looking pretty good over the last few hours.

We checked them while you were sleeping.

Rodney stood up from his seated position and leaned toward me.

I continued lying on the hospital bed.

Little brother, I'm going to take off for a while since you are in the clear.

I left my number at the nurse's station and informed them to call me if you need anything or if they need me.

I love you man

Get some rest.

I will see you later.

I love you to brother

Thank you for hanging out with me.

Rodney left the hospital room while the nurses

we're still attending to my medical needs.

I gazed off in a different direction.

Finally, the nurses were all done.

They exited the room.

I found myself all alone waiting for someone to

enter the room.

All I wanted to hear was Joe you're okay

enough to go home.

That statement never came to fruition for days

yet to come.

My stay in the hospital was very problematic.

I had work to do.

I had a company to run.

I sat there for hours starring at the television. Anything to take my attention off the fact I was confined to the hospital was of interest to me. A nurse entered my room every hour to take my vital signs and update my medical charts. Finally, a doctor entered my room that could provide me with some answers.

The doctor was followed close behind by a group of physicians.

Hi, Joe

I'm Doctor Thomas

These are resident physicians; do you mind if they observe and sit in?

No, it's okay.

The doctor looked me over while the resident physicians followed close behind.

Two or more of everything was occurring.

One stethoscope than another.

One ear view than another ear view.

One nostril gaze than another nostril gaze.

Looking good young fella!

All is in the clear at the present time.

We will be on hourly rounds and stop in every

so often to check on you whether it's me or one

of my doctors.

Don't hesitate to press that call button if you

need us, okay.

Thank you, Doc.

Sounds good!

At this point I was feeling fine.

I wanted him to exit the room and leave me be

just as fast as he entered the room.

I wanted to be alone.

I wanted time to think to myself.

The doctor said his goodbye and exited the

room.

Simultaneously, all the student doctors in

unison said some form of random expression of

goodbye as well.

This Page Intentionally Left Blank

Chapter 4

Collective Fear

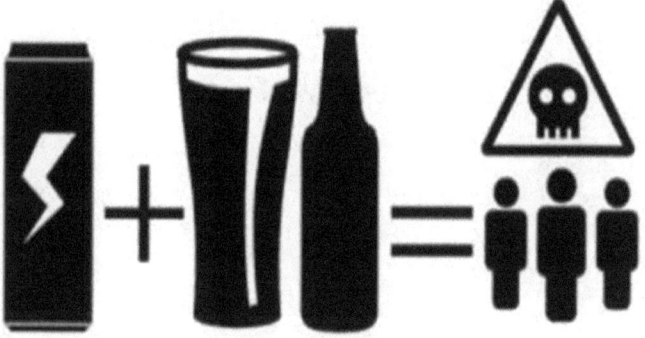

Soon I found myself all alone.

What was I to do?

I laid all by my lonesome in that creepy

hospital room, in that creepy hospital bed.

Negative thoughts started running through my

head as if I was back in the Marine Corp

running through a mine field packed with

explosives.

One explosion after another.

Each sequence of explosions all ended the same

way with death.

To take my mine of those negatives thoughts I

tuned the television to anything, anything that

would detour my mine off dying this day.

www.joevalentine.org

I told myself it was not a good day to die.

The time lapsed at a Snell's pace.

I paid little attention to what was on the tube in front of me.

Television seemed of little interest to me the more and more I thought about escaping from the hospital.

Hours passed by, yet the fear of death had not evaded me.

The fear of death was still very much at the forefront and terrified me enough I could not fall asleep.

The thought of death repeatedly entered and exited my mind.

It is said each of our minds are the dumping grounds for Satan.

It is said it's here where he unloads negative thoughts, plants seeds of doubts, and stakes his flag of lack of faith in the ground of the mind.

It is also said we equally have the power to supersede all the negative thoughts Satan offloads in that mind field called our mind.

This I must have forgotten.

It was here at this moment I was losing the battle and Satan was unloading as much as he could in his dumping grounds, my mind.

I was so afraid to die I remembered thinking at this moment.

As a result, it became my mission to stay awoke if I could.

The Sleep Athlon was on!

Every hour on the half hour a nurse popped through the door.

Each nurse would enter the room with a less than engaging smile on her face.

I don't believe it was my fault for those facial expressions rather the nurses seeing the same old monotony day in and day out repeatedly I imagine was the root cause.

Hi, Joe.

I'm just checking your vitals again.

Do you need anything?

No, I'm okay.

I was a man and it was that manhood that was reluctant to tell the nurse I believed death was standing beside my bed.

So, I said nothing about it and kept my thoughts to myself.

The nurse said some parting words as she prepared to exit the room.

Okay, you just let us know with the ring of the call button or tell one of us during our rounds if you need anything.

I will be going off duty shortly, so another nurse will be taking care of you.

Okay.

The nurse walked out of the room.

I attempted to find something interesting on television as my hospital phone started blowing up with numerous phone calls.

My family called, employees called, my children called, and Rodney called to check and see how I was doing.

During each of these calls I failed to mention I was scared crazy.

I was too scared to go to sleep for fear of death. On the other hand, I cemented that everything was going find and I was on the speedy road to recovery.

Many people made a promise to make their appearance tomorrow after church.

I watched television straight through the night and dozed off a few different times.

Each time I managed to shut my eyes a nurse entered the room to check my vitals and complete her rounds.

Before I knew it, the night had gone.

Night gave away to morning as the Sun came up and showered sunlight into the hospital room. Knock, knock!

Knock, knock I heard a familiar voice say at the door.

I couldn't see around the corner or directly at the door, but I certainly tried to look.

I heard the door slowly open.

The sound of multiple footsteps walking into the room was evident.

Seconds later.

Hey Joe!

Hey Mrs. Shirley!

My face lite up with a smile from ear to ear. My visitor was not my mother Shirley but my

secretary and personal administrative assistant
Mrs. Shirley.

That's what she started out as.

Now she was much more than that to me.

She was my second mother figure who always
expressed sound instructions and guidance to
me. Seeing Mrs. Shirley's face and hearing that
distinctive voice eased my soul and pushed
back those negative thoughts of death.

Not too far behind Mrs. Shirley was the rest of
our corporate management team; Gina, Amber,
Antonio, Connie and Rodney.

It was as if they all started talking all at once.

(Gina): Hey Joe!

(Amber): How are you doing Joe?

(Antonio): Mr. Robinson, how is it going?

(Rodney): I told you brother I would be back!

I sat up in the hospital bed as if to project a strong leadership image.

I don't know how successful I was at that and don't even know why the thought crossed my mind.

Mrs. Shirley and I picked up right where we left off, talking about spirituality, Jesus Christ, God and a purpose driven life.

God isn't through with you yet Joe!

God has some great things for you to do.

I told you, you were anointed.

I can feel it; he is not done with you yet.

Mrs. Shirley always knew the words to inspire and encourage me just as she always inspired her own three sons.

All three of her sons were successful men,
fathers, college athletes, college graduates,
played years in the NFL and men of great faith.
It was that same nurturing I was fortunate
enough to experience from her and her
husband Jerry Sr. who was Iowa All-time
greatest athlete ever.
It was her words that lifted my spirit that day.
We talked about my children, getting well and
hospital food.
Every time I started talking about the office,
Rodney redirected my conversation.
Don't worry about a company, Joe.
A company will take care of itself.

You must get yourself better and stay away
from those energy drinks, so you will be
available to have a company.

Those kids won't their father before they want
a company.

I guess you're right, Rodney.

An hour passed as we fellowshipped and
socialized in the hospital room.

It was time to say our goodbye's.

There was hugs all the way around.

We completed the visit by holding hands and
Mrs. Shirley led us in prayer around my
hospital bed.

I watched and wished I was leaving with them
as everyone left the room.

I was in high spirits and feeling emotionally good.

A few hours alone, I found myself back at the same state fearing falling asleep.

Fearing death.

Chapter 5

Touch Of Compassion

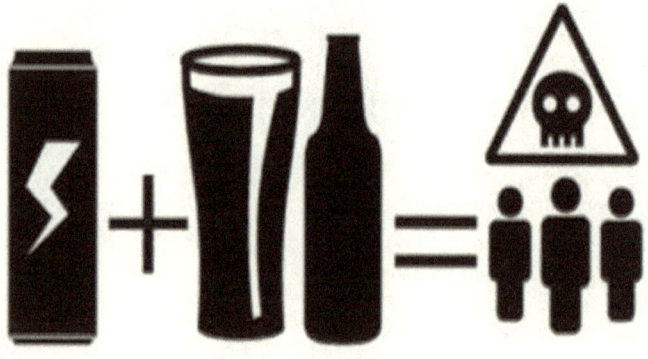

It was getting late into the night. A nurse completed checking my vital signs and exited the room.

I laid there quietly while attempting to watch late night, talk show television.

Sleep started getting the best of me but so was the anxiety of dying.

I tossed and turned.

Finally, I decided to make my final position looking up, laying directly on my back.

I grabbed the television remote and turned the T.V. off.

The room lite up immediately.

It was as if the scenery was right out of a movie.

The dark mid length curtains were parted down the middle.

The split between the two curtains left a gap like the parting of the Red Sea for the moonlight to shine into my room.

The moonlight bounced off the buildings and glared down into the room.

A beam of glowing light pierced in between the curtains.

For a moment all the fear I was internalizing left.

I took in the moment and thought to myself how beautiful the light looked as it came into my room.

I was at peace but then the tranquility departed.

Concern and despair shot through me.

What I thought was all but gone resurfaced

with vengeance!

I spoke aloud to myself and Jesus.

Father, I don't want to die!

God, please let me live!

God, I'm a single father.

Who is going to take care of JoQuan and Jayla

if I die?

Father help me please!

God, allow me to be around for my adult

children and grandchildren!

God, please allow me to complete your purpose

for my life here on Earth!

Father, I haven't fulfilled that promise I made

to you when I was seven.

www.joevalentine.org

Father, please allow me more time to fulfil that promise I made to you!

The dismay I was feeling was on ten.

A scale zero to ten could not go any higher.

I was lying flat on my back.

I stared into the darkest of the room.

Decades earlier near the ripe old age of seven God and I had a conversation.

This conversation occurred while I was on my death bed and is detailed in a book series entitled, "Watchers Angels Are Among Us."

Nevertheless, without warning as I stared into the darkness of the room something happened!

A hand touched me!

An open hand touched me on the topside of my right thigh!

I jumped in astonishment.

I scanned the room with both of my eyes hastily only to see no one here with me.

I said not a word.

I know I wasn't going crazy.

I felt an open hand, four fingers and a thumb resting on my right thigh.

My eyes were wide open as if I could see in the dark. Yet, the moonlight shining into the room provided me with the ability to see.

Nothing or no one was in the room with me.

I was frightened for a split second and even acted out the actions of being terror-stricken but internally afraid I was not.

I turned in the bed to lay on my left side.

I curled into a half ball by pulling my knees towards my chest.

I was facing towards the room door with my back closest to the window.

Unaware of what was yet still to come, this was one time I hoped the nurse stepped through the door to take my vital signs.

Without warning a hand rested itself again on my right thigh.

This time the hand was atop the side of my right thigh due to how I was positioned in the bed.

This time I wasn't scared at the touch on my thigh.

This time I was full of even more inner peacefulness.

This time the touch seemed very familiar.

I knew who it was!

Granddad!!!!!!

I quickly realized the hand touched me literally in the same identical place my grandfather had always touched his grandchildren when he wanted to awake us from sleep.

Granddad would simulate being a fly at times. Sometimes he would use thread and touch our faces and legs all while cracking up as we slapped ourselves to kill the make-believe fly. Other times he would irritate us while sleeping by placing his hand on our right thigh, removing it and placing it back until we woke up.

I can still see the distinctive three horizontal wrinkles at the edge of his eyes when he laughed.

I can still visualize the tears of joy filling up in his eyes from laughing so hard at our expense.

I teared up!

Then I decided to recognize his presence and communicated back to him.

Thank you, Granddad, for letting me know I'm going to be okay!

Thank you for being here with me.

All went back to normal shortly thereafter.

I fell asleep right away free of anymore thoughts and fears of death.

I slept through the entire night.

This was the first time I was not awoken by nurses checking my vital machines or entering and exiting my hospital room since my stay here.

I even slept through breakfast that morning.

Energy drinks nor any other supplement could substitute and make up for my lack of sleep.

I awoke for the first time in months feeling rejuvenated.

It was still early on Monday morning.

I felt pretty good this morning and thought about my parents.

I could only imagine what they are going through after they heard the news that one of their boys was in the hospital with heart troubles.

Then the hospital phone rung.

Surprised as to who was calling me this early in the morning at the hospital, I answered it.

Hello.

Hey, how are you doing?

I heard a familiar comforting voice on the other end.

If no other person loved me or cared about my well-being in the world, I knew this voice did.

I felt like a child who fell and bumped his knee who was waiting to be soothed.

On the other end of the phone was the woman who gave me life and carried me into this world, my mother.

I perked up in the bed and smiled as I heard her voice.

Mom had a tough time raising three boys pretty much on her own.

Father helped but he was in and out of our lives.

She had an even tougher time showing us a display of affection and emotions growing up.

But this time with the lapse of time and the lapse of age came understanding and wisdom.

Mother today was not the mother of yesterday who believed in pure unfiltered tough love.

Today, meaning in recent years mom had evolved.

She evolved into a compassionate, emotional and loving person first.

Hey, son!

How are you doing?

Ma'am, I'm doing just fine.

I stated like a spoiled little kid licking his wounds.

I became overwhelmed with excitement.

I could not wait any longer to tell her of the news.

I wanted her to know her Father Delmar (pronounced Delma) visited me last night.

Mom!

Momma!

Guess what?

What?

Are you okay?

I was so excited to tell her I disregarded her question.

You wouldn't believe what happened to me last night!

Mom sat in silence as if to wait for more bad news about me being hospitalized.

Then she spoke.

Lord don't tell me you have more medical problems!

I will cut my vacation short and head back home immediately!

No, don't cut your vacation short, I'm okay.

But Mom!

But Mom you have to hear this!

Last night, I turned the television off and sat in the dark waiting to fall asleep.

I could tell mother wanted me to get on with the story.

I could hear her take a deep breath as if she was preparing for more bad news.

Come on now, tell me what's going on!

Well, while I was in pitch black, in my room all alone last night I started thinking about dying.

I started thinking about all the things I have not accomplished with my life.

I started thinking about my kids.

I started thinking about all I would miss with my grandkids.

Then it happened!

A hand touched me on my right thigh!

I jumped.

I was surprised but not scared.

Nobody was in the room with me!

Mom sat on the other end of the phone and listened in silence.

I could tell, I had her full attention.

Mother remained in silence as I continued to explain what occurred.

I quickly turned on my left side and curled into a semi ball.

I pulled the hospital blanket over me as if to hide.

Then it happened again.

The open hand touched me on my right thigh again.

Only this time it touched me on the side of my right thigh as if it wanted to comfort me and let me know I was going to be okay!

Before I could explain to mother who or what I thought had touched me on my right thigh with and open hand she started crying.

Then she spoke.

That was DAD!

That was your grandfather!

I know, mom!

That's what I thought immediately after the hand touched me the second time!

Mom responded.

It was granddad!

I know it was him!

Yeah, your grandfather use to grab you kids there all the time, messing with you kids while you were asleep.

He sure did use to crackup laughing as you guys slapped his hand away.

That must have been Dad!

Dad must have been trying to tell you, you were going to be okay.

Yes!

I know it!

Granddad was trying to tell me not to worry about dying right now.

I could hear mom still trying to hold back the tears.

We talked for a while longer about all I had missed this weekend at the 130th Taylor-Jordan family reunion in Rose Hill, Mississippi.

The conversation ended as we said our goodbyes.

Alright, son.

Are you sure you don't want me to head back up north?

No, mom!

I'm okay now.

Alright!

I'm going to let go and let you get some more rest now.

Okay, mom.

Tell everyone hi and that I'm sorry I missed the family reunion.

Everybody already knows.

You just do what those doctors are telling you to do.

Everyone down here at the family reunion said to tell you we are praying for you.

The entire family has prayed for you.

I love you son.

I've already told the nurses and the doctors to call me if anything, anything at all happens to you.

Alright mom, I love you too.

I'll talk with you later.

Bye.

I could hear mom sniffling and holding back the tears about her father visiting me as she hung up the telephone.

I also imagine some of that sniffling was because drinking energy drinks almost killed her son.

In the days to follow many visitors made their way to Allen Hospital just to see me.

I appreciated the visits nevertheless; I wasn't looking forward to them.

I was looking forward to getting off the third floor and getting out of the hospital.

Stacy the childhood friend and nurse I called at the outset of this medical debacle took care of me several days I was hospitalized.

Seeing a familiar face daily really made my day.

Her mere presence made my stay at the hospital much easier.

Midweek there was a soft knock at my door.

I wasn't expecting any additional visitors I thought to myself.

Suddenly, the door pushed open with force.

I heard the little pitter patty of feet running towards me.

I could not see who it was on the other side of the curtain separating my view from the hospital room door.

Then I heard a long drown out

Dadddddddddy!!

It was my youngest child, my daughter.

Daddy!

I lit up with the biggest smile on my face.

I knew that little squeaky voice anywhere.

My daughter was six years old but going on the old ripe age of thirty in her mind.

I knew she missed my presence just as I missed hers.

Worrying about my young six-year-old was one of my biggest concerns while I was housed in the hospital.

I often wondered how she was holding on in my absence over the last few days.

I wondered was she terrified in the middle of the night.

Every and I mean every night between the hours of 1 and 2 a.m. my daughter would awake, leave her own bedroom and search the house for me.

Most nights she would arise from her sleep and walk down the hallway making her way into my room. She and her brother six years her elder had been in my custody since she was two years old.

This energy drink debacle almost robbed me of the opportunity to enjoy all of my children.

Hey, little lady!

Hey, Daddy!!!!

She ran and jumped on top of the silver railing running down the side of my bed.

I grabbed her by the shoulders and pulled her up into the bed.

She gave me the biggest hug and I gave her the biggest hug right back.

I could have missed out on these loving interactions if the energy drinks would have won a few days ago.

At the bat of an eye my twelve-year-old son walked around the long tan full length curtain.

He was closely followed by someone I wasn't expecting to see my ex, the kids' mother.

Hey, Dad!

Hey, son!

The kids' mother and I had very little words to say to one another since the end of our thirteen-year relationship, but she spoke.

I thought I'd bring them to see you.

Thank you!

Thank you for bringing them.

The kids were very inquisitive.

They asked all types of questions about the wires, cords and machines hooked up to me.

Most of all they wanted to know was I going to be okay.

They wanted to know when they were coming back home.

My heart melted.

They wanted to be home with me just as much as I wanted to be back at home with them.

The only thing that stood between that happening was my ongoing usage of energy drinks.

An hour later we had to say our tearful goodbye's.

It's time for us to go, tell your father goodbye.

Bye Dad.

My six-year-old daughter on the other hand had other plans.

Daddy I don't want to go.

I want to stay here with you.

Sweetie, you can't stay with me.

Dad will be home in a few days.

No Daddy, I want to stay, please!

My daughter started tearing up and crying.

I started tearing up and crying along with her.

Darn, energy drinks!

You must go with your mother.

You guys will stay with her until I get out of the hospital!

Please, Daddy I want to stay with you.

No sweetie you can't.

My heart broke.

It tormented me to watch her cry and scream.

She wanted to stay by my side.

After a few minutes of convincing she agreed to leave with her mother without further confrontation.

My family left and I was left lying in a hospital bed regretting the day I put an energy drink up to my lips.

I couldn't wait to be released from the hospital to tell everyone I cared about of the dangers I encountered by drinking energy drinks and high doses of caffeine.

Chapter 6

Lone Star Death

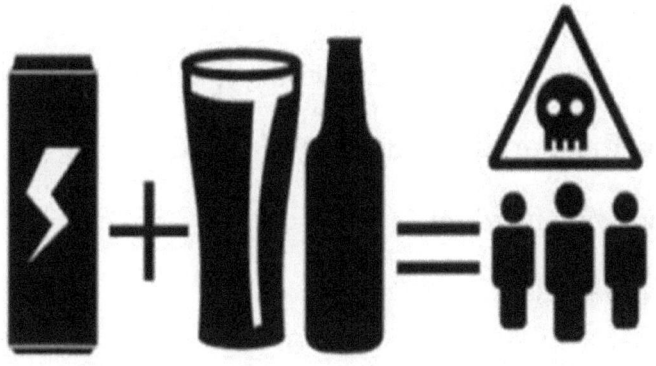

www.joevalentine.org

A week passed by. The day of discharge finally came. The care I received at Allen Hospital was second to none, compassionate, caring, professional and spot on the morning of my arrival into the emergency room.

Nonetheless, I was eager to go.

I wanted out of here.

It took a few hours before the doctor signed off on my discharge papers.

Not a minute to soon I was off in a wheelchair enroute to the street level where I would exit the hospital.

Finally, my truck pulled up with my friend driving it.

The nurse helped me out of the wheelchair and into the passenger seat even though I felt I did not need her help.

I clamped the seatbelt in and off we went.

This was the first time I saw and felt the sunlight on my skin in several days.

After a few minutes we arrived in my neighborhood near my home.

My home was literally two blocks down a small hill from my older brothers' home.

I desperately wanted to see him, so we stopped by.

He just arrived back in town from our family reunion down south of the Mason and Dixon Line a few hours earlier.

Pulling up to my brothers' home I noticed several vehicles and friends from our childhood standing in the driveway talking.

Some were talking, some were working on their vehicles.

Once we came to a complete stop, I exited the truck.

I walked towards the driveway and turned to walk down it in the direction of the garage.

A burgundy Hummer that I knew all too well was sitting in the reversed position in the driveway. The doors and the rear hatch of the Hummer were wide open.

A childhood friend, like a big brother to me was

installing televisions throughout his Hummer.

I approached Terrance's Hummer from the

passenger side door.

I was yearning to tell him where I had been.

I looked inside the front of the Hummer but

did not see Terrance.

However, in the cup holder in between the

seats I saw an unopened grey and blue can.

It was an energy drink waiting to be consumed.

I took a few more steps past the passenger

door.

I stopped at the passenger rear door.

Terrance was sitting in the rear driver side seat

twisting red, green and yellow wires together

over his head as a large television dangled in the air.

I spoke to him.

What's up bro?

What's up Joe Rob?

Man, I'm trying to get these TV's installed in my Hummer before it gets to cold.

Your brother told me you were in the hospital. Did you just get out?

Yep, they finally let me go.

Bro, did you know why I was in there?

Your brother told me something was wrong with your heart, right?

Yes, but do you know why something was wrong with my heart?

Before Terrance could reply, I replied for him.

My heart went into overdrive because of one of those energy drinks like you have in your cup holder upfront!

Those things are terrible for you brother.

I almost killed myself drinking them.

You might want to stop drinking them Terrance.

I'm good brother don't worry about me.

I've been drinking energy drinks a long time with no problems.

That is the problem Terrance, me too, I had no problems until there was a problem!

Energy drinks keep me woke at night while I'm at work.

I need them brother, third shift at John Deere's is not a joke!

I drink one before I go in to work and I drink one during my shift in the middle of the night.

They keep me going!

They give me the energy I need.

I could see it was no convincing him to stop drinking energy drinks, but I had to try.

I explained to Terrance what happened in detail and he looked disinterested as if it could not happen to him.

I finally gave up on this endless conversation that wasn't making much of a difference.

I gave Terrance one last message pertaining to energy drinks.

Just be careful!

Terrance replied.

I'm good little brother, now come around here and hold this T.V. up for me.

I leaned inside the passenger rear door and pushed the television up towards the ceiling of the Hummer while Terrance bolted down the screws into the brackets mounted to the ceiling.

After a few minutes we were all done.

We said our goodbye that day and gave each other a hug with a normal pat on the back.

Months later, a mutual friend informed me Terrance quit his job at Deere and Company and opted to move out of the state.

Terrance moved to Dallas in pursuit of a better life and to evade the Iowa frigid winters.

One spring afternoon, I logged into Facebook.

I generally minded my own business and steered clear of viewing news feeds.

I wanted no parts of other people's drama, cheating, arguing, accusations, infidelities, daily relationship changes, family feuds, toxicity and dysfunction.

This login was different.

I was drawn to view my news feed.

At first glimpse I saw it!

I spoke to myself out loud.

No!!!

No!!!

There must be a mistake!

The more I scrolled down the more post I saw from other people's news feeds.

This can't be!

Instinctively, I thought to reach out on Facebook to someone who would know the answer to what I was reading on my news feed.

Hesitantly, I scrolled the cursor up to the Facebook search line.

I typed in Terrance's brother's name Todd and his page populated.

I was terrified to ask!

I didn't want to ask!

I did not want it to be true.

I opened Facebook Messenger.

I sent Todd a message.

Todd, is Terrance okay?

Tell me what I'm seeing on Facebook isn't true!

Todd responded.

It's true.

He's gone!

Something happened to his heart.

Mom and I are on our way to Dallas now!

My heart dropped in my chest.

Oh my God!

I didn't know what to say.

I was numb.

I sat there in silence.

I sat there like I didn't hear what I just heard.

No one had to tell me what it was that caused Terrance's heart to go into overdrive.

I already knew.

Maybe I was wrong, but I had a pretty good idea what it was.

The vision of the energy drink sitting in his Hummer's cup holder resonated in my head.

I'm sure energy drinks had a role in it.

Who would have known that would be the last time I'd see Terrance alive?

I thought about all the things Terrance was going to miss.

This perfectly healthy man who worked out often was now gone.

Was he gone because God called him home or was, he gone because of his own freewill to drink energy drinks aided in his departure?

Empty energy drink bottles were found in his trash can and scrolled throughout his apartment.

Chapter 7

I Would Have Missed

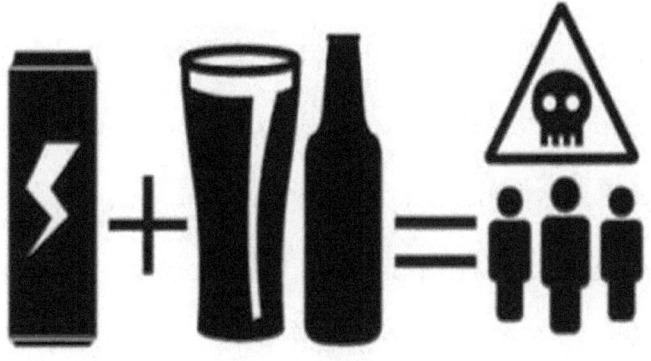

www.joevalentine.org

My focus shifted from my friend. It shifted to thinking about my own run ins with high doses of caffeine and energy drinks. My near catastrophe had it gone the other way would have been a disaster for me.

My near catastrophe would have been devastating to my children, my brothers, my mother, my father, my friends and many other loved ones just as my friend Terrance's passing was to me and his family.

Hundreds if not thousands of people would have been left hurt, confused and questioning what happened.

No one wants to ever receive that personal notification that a loved one has died although we know those notifications will happen sooner or later.

No one wants to stop by a friend or loved one's home for a visit only to find that loved one has died from a cardiac arrest.

If this occurred, immediately from the shock and trauma one would be experiencing one would never contemplate nor investigate whether that loved one was a victim of high doses of caffeine.

The surprise, astonishment or devastation from the ongoing happenstance would most likely lead you to believe it just was the deceased persons time to go.

This prompted me to contemplate my own life.

Then I thought about all the things I would have missed if I had not survived.

What would I have missed if I died that September day?

Who would have spoken up for me?

Who would have told my story?

Who would have told the world of my terrifying experience caused by drinking energy drinks?

There would have been NOBODY!

Nobody would have known.

Nobody would have spoken up for me.

Nobody would have told this story.

Nobody would have told of this experience and my encounter with energy drinks.

That voice would have been silenced had I died that day, in that emergency room.

I would have missed the birth of my grandchildren.

I would have missed the accolades in sports of my sons.

I would have missed the spiritual progress of my brother.

I would have missed the experience and rebirth of myself spiritually.

I would have missed the graduation of my daughter receiving her master's degree.

I would have missed the new friendships I've gained since moving to the coast.

I would have missed my son's basketball games in high school.

I would have missed attending science projects at my daughters' school.

I would have missed my grandson eating my French fries with me.

I would have missed dancing and singing with my granddaughters.

I would have missed cooking and barbecuing with my grandson my greatest helper.

I would have missed my grandson crying the night I was to leave Huntsville to go back home to Boston, which confirmed I was loved.

I would have missed the in-depth conversations with my daughter in laws.

I would have missed the numerous emails and instant messages I've received over the years from readers of my Facebook daily Midday

Motivational post wherein I'm told my words make a difference in somebody's day.

What will you miss if you continue scarfing down energy drinks like there is no tomorrow?

Ironically, there will be no tomorrow if you have an adverse reaction.

Have you thought about that?

Probably not because until this happened to me, I had not thought about it either.

Have you thought about your numbers being called in the energy drink lottery and you have an adverse reaction?

God forbid you take a drink of an energy drink and it becomes your last drink.

Some will say, "But I have no adverse reaction to energy drinks!"

And to that I say, neither did I.

Neither did I, at first but the constant adjusting

of my heartbeat, up and down, up and down

sooner or later took its toll.

CNN health published an article entitled,

"What the energy drink can do to your body" by

Jacqueline Howard warning us of the potential

dangers of energy drinks.

"They may pose danger to public health,"

warns the World Health Organization.

Children "should not consume" them, cautions

the American Academy of Pediatrics.

You will always find studies and organizations

to support whichever stance you want to take

pertaining to energy drinks.

The American Beverage Association stands by the safety of energy drinks, indicating that many of their ingredients are also found in common foods and have been rigorously studied for safety. Whichever stance you take whether for energy drinks or against energy drinks neither report will do you any good if your dead or laying on an operating table from drinking energy drinks.

This Page Intentionally Left Blank

Chapter 8

Under The Knife

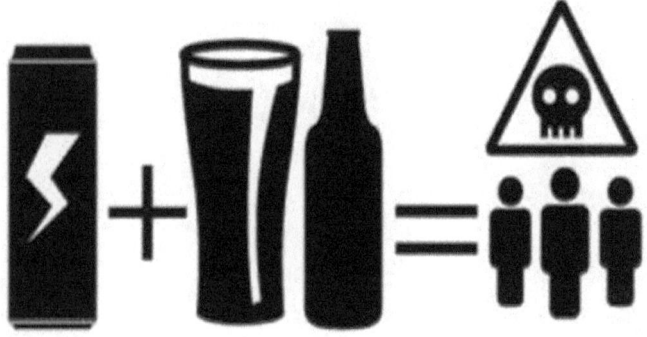

Amonth later I found myself laying on an operating table. I was inside a hospital surgery room.

The heart doctor I was seeing following the energy drink encounter scheduled me for a heart procedure.

The heart procedure was to correct the damage done as a result of my heart beating nearly 250 beats per minute.

The operating room felt lonely and very cold. The hospital gown did little to warm me up.

Two nurses guided the surgical table I was lying on into the center of the room.

They placed me under intense lights that started warming my body up.

I knew the lights weren't specifically for me. The lights I imagine were for the surgeon's sight during my heart procedure.

The surgeon assistants surrounded me and prepared me for surgery.

I starred up at the bright lights.

A male surgeon assistant stepped up on the raised surgical floor next to the table I was laying on.

How is it going young fella?

I starred at the surgical assistant because I was in no mood for small talk.

I was already terrified about the procedure and now this guy wanted to casually talk as if we

were walking down the Boardwalk on Venice
Beach.

I said nothing.

I said nothing at least not at first.

The male surgical assistant spoke.

Not talking much today.

Well, were going to take good care of you
anyway.

You my friend are very lucky.

Somebody on the other side was looking out for
you.

Most people who come into emergency rooms
across America in your condition never leave.

He piqued my curiosity, so I decided to open
my mouth and converge with him.

Why is that?

Because they generally are already dead!

That wasn't the response I was expecting to hear.

The look on my face surely said the same.

The male surgeon was very talkative and continued to inform me how dangerous energy drinks were to the human body.

Most of the people we see in here for this procedure have some effects from some form of energy supplement.

Many people especially athletes and college students come in here with their hearts in overdrive from drinking energy drinks or high doses of caffeine.

Most people do not know energy drinks can speed up the heart to the point of death.

You my friend I consider one of the lucky ones.

This procedure and staying away from energy drinks should provide you with the opportunity to live a long productive life.

Don't worry, we will get you all fixed up.

Shortly, a nurse will come over and give you some anesthesia that will put you to sleep.

When you awake you will be all fixed?

Moments later a mask covered my face and I was out.

I awoke a few hours later and ultimately discharged from my one-day inpatient procedure.

I was discharged from the hospital with a lifetime supply and reoccurring medication prescriptions and ongoing scheduled doctor appointments to monitor my heart.

This was one cause and effect of years of downing energy drinks and intaking high doses of caffeine.

This was my new reality.

This was something I had to come to grips with.

Years of usage and years of energy drink abuses had taken a toll on my heart.

I like so many others have purchased energy drinks in bulk and multiple packs to keep them on hand.

Energy drinks were my substitute for sleep.

Energy drinks became my nutrients and my vegetables.

Energy drinks were my number one substitute choice for energy.

Energy drinks became my very own substitute prescription for Viagra.

Playing basketball and in need of a boost during the game, an energy drink minutes prior was my answer.

Energy drinks became my legal drug of choice.

Sick, no problem.

I drunk an energy drink to give me an energy boost.

Semi-Pro football game, no problem.

I drunk an energy drink and rarely got tired during the game. I could run and tackle all day.

Sex, no problem.

I drunk an energy drink and could go for hours never getting tired.

No sleep, no problem.

A few energy drinks woke me right up.

Drained from hours of service to my country, patrolling, hiking, marching, running in the United States Marine Corp, no problem.

A few energy drinks did the trick and boosted me right up.

Most people today has forgone the traditional ways of recapturing rest and getting sleep.

It is now common to function on a few hours of sleep.

Many people are working two and three jobs just to make ends meet.

Many people are working full time jobs and attending college to make a better life for themselves and their families.

Many people are juggling work, juggling after school sporting events, academic events, clubs, and / or societies and many other events their children participate in.

These activities all need energy and many millions of people daily find that energy in the form of energy drinks or high doses of caffeine for a pick me up.

Extreme pressure is on most people for a pick me up.

Some find there pick me up by way of coffee.

Some find there pick me up by way of drugs.

Some find there pick me up by way of energy drinks.

Some are seeking any type of energy stimuli, so they can make it through the day or make it through the night without a hiccup or misstep in completing the task or job that's at hand.

Society today is hell bent on finding quick solutions.

We want quick solutions for financial success.

We want quick solutions for educational achievement.

If most of us could we would skip being a college Freshman and jump to be a college graduate, graduating with the degree prior to doing the hard work.

We often have these desires of receiving a reward without doing the work.

This mentality of quick solutions is seen all over society in just about every aspect including gaining energy.

College student athletes no longer want to attend college but would prefer to jump straight to the professional leagues.

Many want the new car without the new car payments.

Many want the beautiful relationships or marriage without the disagreements or moments of dysfunction.

Many want the pot of gold without first seeing the rainbow.

Millions want to feel great all day without putting the right nutrients in our bodies. Millions want to lose weight without eating right and exercising so many people continue to search for the super diet of all super diets. Millions want our tanks to be full of energy without making deposits into the sleep bank.

Nothing substitutes sleep and eating right!

Our creator made us that way.

He even documented it and outlined a natural remedy for us in his words he left behind in the Bible.

In the Bible or in most religious books you will find something referencing sleeping, eating and dieting right.

The Bible states the following;

Daniel 1:12 (New International Version),

"Please test your servants for ten days: Give us nothing but vegetables to eat and water to drink.

Another scripture from the Bible reads as follows.

Daniel 1:15 (New International Version), "At the end of the ten days they looked healthier and better nourished than any of the young men who ate the royal food."

I'm sure some similar messages appear in other religious doctrines.

We are uniquely made.

We are made to solve our own problems.

We are made to refill our own energy banks and no energy stimuli is needed.

For every deposit of sleep, we put in, we get a return and boost of energy withdrawal we can take out.

There is no quick fix.

There is no quick solution without having some profound or traumatic effects.

In the theory of cause and effect, the universal law states for every effect there is or will be a definite cause.

Likewise, for every cause there is and will be a definite effect.

Every one of our behaviors and actions will create and effect that will manifest in our lives sooner or later.

Energy and rest is no different.

Energy drinks was my cause and one effect is now living on a lifetime supply of medications that help control the speed of my heart rate.

Energy drinks was my cause and another effect is now lifelong medical bills stacking up.

For every cause there will be an equal and opposite effect.

You can't continue to drink energy drinks and expect nothing will happen just because it has not happened yet.

Everybody has different effects because each of us are made different.

Some will have immediate effects.

Some will have effects months or years from now.

Some won't have effects at all and will be perfectly fine.

I myself thought I was in the latter category.

I thought energy drinks and high doses of caffeine would have no bad effect on me.

You know your body better than I do.

I thought I knew my body as well until it happened to me.

That day my heart went into overdrive after drinking energy drinks was something I never contemplated.

I bet you are not contemplating it either.

It was something so far removed from my mind it was not on my radar.

If you are drinking energy drinks or high doses of caffeine, make yourself aware of the risk.

Life presents us with choices.

Often those choices have some risk and those choices have some rewards.

The energy drink industry has made it their business, literally their business to take that risk and reward opportunity with your life.

This Page Intentionally Left Blank

Chapter 9

Why Are You Surprised

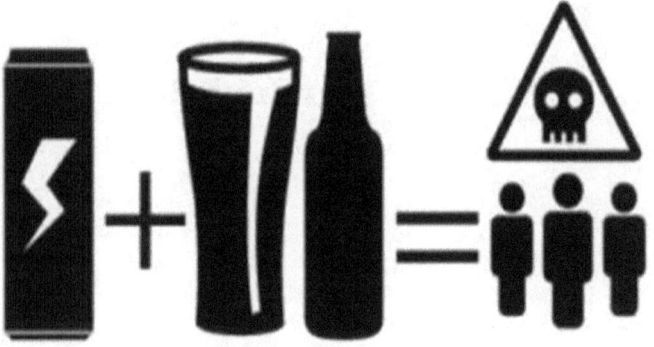

Why do you look so surprised that such a product is for sale in the United States? The energy drink and caffeine beverage business is a global commodity all across the world. However, in the United States like most countries there are many questionable products offered for sale on our grocery store shelves and most Americans are not aware of it. There are questionable products in our foods, in our beverages and even in the feed we feed to our animals we later consume.

The U.S. does limit questionable or possibly dangerous ingredients that may be needed in a product to consumable levels.

This means the levels are consumable but still may cause long term side effects.

This would be no different than pouring water into your oil in your vehicle or water into your gas tank and expecting no real damage to be done.

This means filling up your car or S.U.V. that runs off unleaded gas with diesel gas and expecting no real damage to be done.

Energy drinks is one of those items that also could be questionable but allowed into the U.S. Market.

Some of you may say the government would not allow questionable items into the U.S. Market. Contrary to U.S. citizens belief the

U.S. has allowed numerous items into our homes throughout the U.S. history.

I'm sure with a little research you can find a number of household products approved by our government in your home right now that could be hazardous to your health if used in large quantities.

Coca-Cola utilized cocaine as an ingredient from 1886 to 1929.

Today the U.S. government has allowed opioids into the U.S. Market all well knowing all opioids contain an illegal drug in it called heroin.

Sure, there are other dangerous items in our food, our meats, our medicines and in our beverages that contain dangerous additives, ingredients or components.

The longevity of shelf life for food and beverage products didn't just occur on there on.

The longevity was created in a lab.

Did you know most blue things you eat, and drink contain chemicals that cause very bad things to our body yet there approved for consumption in the U.S.?

Did you know most yellow colors like in our mac and cheese is dangerous for consumption in large doses?

Did you know most red dyes we see on some of our favorite candy's or in our energy drinks are dangerous to the body in large amounts of consumption.

I'm sure many of you reading this will say just has I did, "but there so good."

Yes, they are good, but the ingredients are also dangerous in large doses.

Due to the ongoing popularity of energy drinks articles and reports outlining potential health risks has been on the rise.

However, these articles are not brought to the forefront by our news media.

These articles are usually small articles tucked under leading headlines.

Some potential risk we overlook is the excessive consumption warnings by the energy drink industry. Often these warnings are in small prints, or ten second postings at the bottom of the screen during advertisement ads.

Caffeine overdose can lead to some real-life medical emergencies.

Palpitations of the heart can result, and this is what I experienced.

Type 2 diabetes can result from too many energy drinks.

High blood pressure, nausea and vomiting, poor dental, stillbirths, convulsions, late term miscarriages, obesity, neurological system problems, cardiovascular system concerns and even death all can be a side-effect of high doses of caffeine or high consumptions of energy drinks.

Mixing energy drinks with another energy drink is like putting money down on a roulette table where your chances of losing your bet is extremely high.

Only your betting your life.

Mixing energy drinks is extremely dangerous.

An even worse risk is mixing energy drinks with alcohol.

Too much caffeine has consequences.

A 16-year-old high school student who was against taking drugs or doing anything illegal collapsed during class at school. He later died from drinking caffeine laced drinks within a two-hour period. His father later said, "It wasn't a car crash that took his life, instead, it was an energy drink."

A 38-year-old male drunk numerous energy drinks and his heart went into cardiac arrest.

After several attempts to get the man stabilized, he died one hour later. The doctors in the Emergency Room said they never seen anything like it.

Many people will not experience some of the above health risk nevertheless, there will be those who will.

Chapter 10

What Is Your Life Worth?

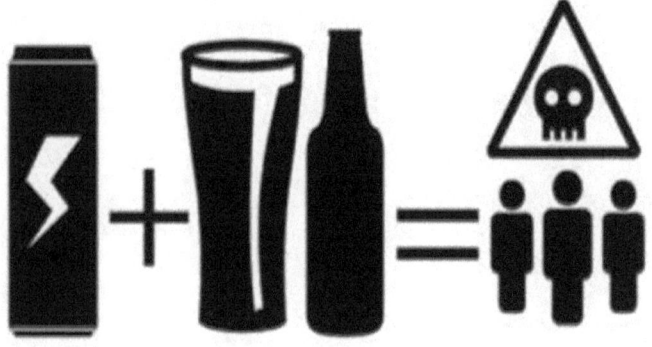

Have you every put a dollar amount on your life? How much is your life worth? How much money will you be willing to die for?

You do realize you will not have the ability to enjoy whatever dollar amount you come up with but who cares?

Somebody else will get to enjoy that dollar amount on your behalf is pretty much what the energy drink industry is saying.

And from the sounds of it the record energy drink annual profits is well worth the payout if an untimely, unexpected, unanticipated death occur on your behalf.

Simply put, the energy drink industry is big business.

The global energy drink market was worth over $39 Billion dollars in 2013.

Furthermore, because people like you or someone you know continues to consume energy drinks in large amounts the industry continues to grow at an accelerated rate.

It has been predicted the global energy drink market will reach $61 Billion dollars near 2020.

It is good business if you are on the receiving end as an investor, stockholder, distributor, manufacturer, delivery driver, employee or indirect benefactor.

Nevertheless, good business for the industry doesn't mean it's good for you.

The industry has evolved into a staple in our society.

We see energy drinks everywhere.

We see energy drinks on countertops at gas stations.

We see energy drinks nuzzled cozily next to other soft drink products in fast-food facilities.

We see energy drinks being given away as samples inside retail outlets.

We turn on the television to watch the Olympics and what do you know!

Energy drink logos and advertisement posters are everywhere.

Venues are covered by energy drink sponsors.

Helmets, skis, clothing, gloves, hats, sunglasses, jackets, socks, shoes, billboards, walls, flags, ground surfaces, swim wear, balls and even in the air overhead you might see energy drink advertisement.

We see energy drinks adoring our coveted athletes' uniforms.

Try to watch a professional sporting event, football, baseball, soccer, hockey or any sport and monitor the time laps before your eyes catch sight of advertisement from an energy drink or caffeinated beverage company.

It will not be long before you see it.

We can't get away from seeing energy drink advertisements.

Energy drink advertising is everywhere.

Energy drink advertising and marketing has taken on a life of it's on.

Energy drinks have taken a great leap in our society.

Some of these companies sponsor racing series, professional athletes, and even collegiate athletic events such as bowl games, and tournaments.

Today we encounter energy drink ads that target college students and youth sporting events.

Everywhere I look I see energy drinks.

I spot them in the checkout line of the world's largest retailer.

I spot them appearing digitally at college sporting events.

I spot them in most workout gyms.

Today you can't take a few steps into a gym without noticing the energy drink coolers, flyers, posters and marketing of the organization's favorite energy drink.

Just about everybody is thirsty to make a profit from the energy drink industry.

Energy drink companies maximize their new-found fame.

These companies pay marketing companies millions of dollars annually to build their brands with the intent to attract the next generation of energy drinkers.

Whether your drinking an energy drink that uses a name with time in it, an energy drink that uses a name with an animal in it, an energy drink that uses a reference to a character in a horror flick all of them may and the key word is may be dangerous to your health.

Do not ignore the numerous warnings in journals and articles published every year.

Is it worth a few energy drink related deaths per year to energy drink companies?

You and I may say no it isn't.

However, the energy drink industry may silently take another stance.

Millions of dollars of profit annually certainly may change a few minds as long as it's not their loved one dying.

The world energy drink market is valued well over 40 billion dollars today.

The industry is very lucrative.

Energy drink sales are anticipated to grow 4 – 5 % in the coming years.

The key categories in the energy drink market are; energy drinks and energy shots neither of which are better than good old-fashioned vegetables and sleep.

To make it more confusing for consumers some energy drinks are labeled as dietary supplements.

This leads many to believe the items will help you lose weight and not be of any harm to you and most of the time this may be true.

But most of the time is not good enough when your life is on the line.

One time for most people is all it takes.

One bad experience may be deadly.

I was one of the lucky ones who survived and had a supernatural helping hand that provided me comfort.

Life is risk and reward.

Risk and reward in the energy drink and caffeine beverage industry is more common than you think.

What if you died after drinking an energy drink or a high dose of caffeine?

Would anyone know that an energy drink or high dose of caffeine may have been the assailant?

What if it takes minutes, hours or days for your heart to go into overdrive after drinking an energy drink or a high dose of caffeine?

What if you have already disposed of the energy drink can or bottle?

Who would know what happened to you?

The Coroner might figure it out after your already deceased and laying on the cold metal table if you're lucky enough.

That luck isn't for you, your luck ran out because at this point, you're already dead.

Rather that luck pertains to the family left behind.

Someone may find the root cause of your heart catastrophe before cremating or putting you into the ground.

This then may start a legal process against a particular energy drink or high caffeinated beverage company.

Your family members may find themselves tangled in a wide web of ongoing legal battles for years to come long after your gone.

Years or even decades down the road the energy drink or high caffeinated beverage company may offer your family a settlement.

Your family members still fighting on your behalf may find themselves in a number of peculiar situations.

Some will be broken mentally from the loss of you.

Some will be shattered financially from ongoing legal fees.

Some will be mentally drained from numerous motions and court hearings.

Not to mention the monstrous remaining legal bill waiting in the shadows from the legal team working extremely hard on your family's behalf.

When all is said and done your life will be worth a few cents on the dollar all while energy drink companies will continue to bring in billions of dollars annually.

Is the risk and reward beneficial to you or to the energy drink industry?

Is it a win, win for you and your family?

I say not.

It's a win, win for the government and taxes.

It is a win, win for the energy drink industry.

It is a win, win for the caffeinated drink industry.

It is a win, win for the average consumer because they get the energy boost, they need.

It is not a win, win for that one consumer that has a bad reaction to consuming to much caffeine.

Energy drink companies will not stop as long as they are making the all mighty dollar.

A recent energy drink commercial I saw on television the other day said the energy drink will give you wings.

I agree.

I agree it will give you your very own set of spiritual wings sooner than you may want to have them.

This Page Intentionally Left Blank

Chapter 11

Under Educated

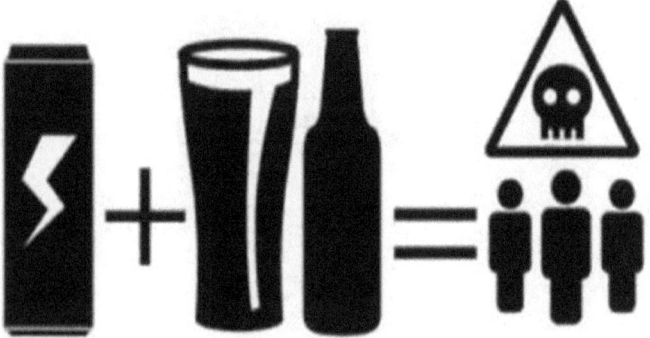

Like most of you guzzling down one energy drink after another we lack education and substance on what we put into our bodies.

I was unaware of the numerous catastrophic possibilities and damage energy drinks and high doses of caffeine could cause to my heart and body.

If you don't believe me just stop in at your local emergency room or doctor's office.

Try asking a Cardiologist or heart specialist that has not been funded or paid by the energy drink industry.

Like anything you will find some that will attest energy drinks do little harm.

Some might even state energy drinks are good for you for its specific purpose, energy or dietary supplement.

You will find some with the strong belief energy drinks should be outlawed for sale in the states and worldwide.

Nevertheless, as long as there is a profitable industry and a dollar to be made the debate good versus bad will continue regardless of most health experts' warnings of the dangers of caffeinated and energy drinks.

You ultimately make the decision of what to put into your body.

Let's weigh the options.

Energy drink companies make millions of dollars annually.

You make a quick unexpected exit to the grave leaving behind your loved ones.

Your loved ones if they are fortunate to prove energy drinks were the direct cause will pursue the energy drink or high dose caffeinated beverage company at fault.

The energy drink company law team will argue the energy drink company is not at fault.

They will argue you the dead individual had freewill and a choice to make.

They will argue you made your choice and that choice was to consume high doses of caffeinated energy drinks.

They will argue you read the warning on the exterior of the energy drink packaging.

They will argue they met government requirements with the compliance of the added warning label to packaging and the small print at the bottom of your television screen during the energy drink television commercials.

After years of legal arguments, years of legal expenses your family might be ready to throw in the towel and enter into a settlement.

You're not happy because your dead and gone. Your family is not happy because not only are they missing you, but very little monies are left after taxes and legal expenses are paid from the settlement.

The energy drink company will present an image of compassion and concern in the public view and might even give back donations annually to selected communities as part of their social responsibility.

If you die as a result of consuming to many energy drinks or too much caffeine rest assured energy drink companies will continue making millions of dollars as if you never existed.

That my friend is what we call capitalism.

That my friend is what we consider a free choice democracy.

Any volunteers?

Who wants to take heart medications for the rest of their life?

Who wants to visit the Cardiologist monthly?

I want to work out, but I question if it's safe to do so.

If you or someone you know continues to drink energy drinks or high doses of caffeine you or even them might be okay and never experience a problem.

I was lucky.

On the other hand, you might be that one person who is not so lucky.

You may not be as fortunate as I was to survive an energy drink induced heart that was racing like a horse on the final leg of the Kentucky Derby.

I only wanted a boost of energy and to return home to my family safe and sound no different than a law enforcement officer beginning his or her shift.

I wanted my energy boost and to live to see another day.

One energy drink is "NO" better than the other.

I'm just and everyday Joe telling you about my own energy drink and high dose of caffeine experience.

This is only my experience with caffeinated beverages and energy drinks.

Just as the energy drink and caffeinated beverage industry warning label that was my warning label to you.

My warning to you was the sharing of my experience.

My experience may not be the average experience with energy drinks and high doses of caffeine but yet it still was an experience I had that very much well could happen to you.

I pray that my experience does not end up being your adventure.

Ultimately, it is your choice what goes into your body and your choice alone.

I've done my job and made you aware, of my experience with energy drinks.

Now, it's your job to continue to play Russian Roulette with your life every time you drink an energy drink or consume high doses of caffeine.

It is your choice to put the gun down and play Russian Roulette no more or continue to take chances assuming nothing will happen as I once did.

The bullet may not be in front of the firing pin this bottle.

The bullet may not be in front of the firing pin this can.

The bullet may not be in front of the firing pin this pill.

The bullet may not be in front of the firing pin this injection, but rest assured the bullet is still in the firing chamber every time you put a caffeinated beverage or energy drink up to your mouth.

If it fires it will be your family and loved ones singing that sad song sooner, then they should have.

Some will say your death was of natural causes because nobody thought to pay attention to the empty energy drink bottles in your wastebasket.

Nobody thought to pay attention to the scattered energy drink or high caffeine induced beverage cans or bottles all over your apartment, house, gym bag or automobile.

It took my bout with energy drinks to realize there is no substitute for water, exercise, a good diet, and a good night's sleep.

Don't just take my word for it.

Do your own research.

Search Google, Bing, YouTube or whatever your search engine preference is for excessive caffeine usage or bad energy drink encounters online.

See the effects for yourself.

Drinking energy drinks caught up with me and it may very well catch up with you if you don't change some habits and learned behaviors.

I did not write this memoir of my experience to discourage you from drinking energy drinks or doses of caffeine.

I wrote this to bring to your attention that the dose and amount of caffeine and energy drinks you consume does matter.

The amount you consume in a given time period can be hazardous to your health.

If you are going to drink energy drinks or high doses of caffeine drink in moderation, drinking in moderation may be beneficial to some and not beneficial to others.

Unfortunately, I was one of the others, so I avoid it all together.

Warning

Don't Ever Mix Energy Drinks With Alcohol or
Another Energy Drink, It Could Be a Cocktail
Mix You Want Recover From!

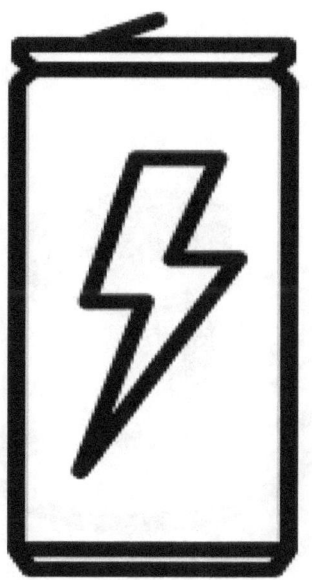

Don't Forget To Share Your Stories With Us!

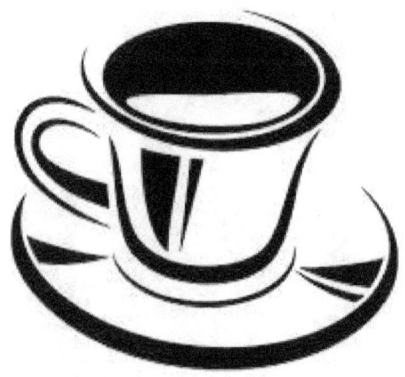

If you're going to consume doses of caffeine and energy drinks, do it safely and with caution.

<u>Other Books Written By This Author</u>

"Watchers, Angels Are Among Us", Book Series

"The Day Energy Drinks Almost Killed Me"

"Midday Motivations, Food For Your Soul"

"UOP, University of Phoenix My Experience"

"Life After MTV's 16 And Pregnant, My New

Reality" – Co-Authored by Isaiah T. Robinson

"Sidelined For Life, Memoirs of Collegiate Athlete

Devin Robinson"

"15 Minute CEO"

Visit Us Online:

www.joevalentine.org

or

Amazon Books.com